MORRIS GREEN

ESSENTIAL

NURSING SKILLS

54 Guides for Nursing Practice

TABLE OF CONTENT

INTRODUCTION

Nurses are the unsung heroes in the complex web of healthcare, bringing compassion, knowledge, and commitment to every patient interaction. Nursing is fundamentally about the deep abilities and attributes that nurses bring to the bedside, not merely about the white coats and antiseptic surroundings. Nursing is a job that requires a complex fusion of technical skill, emotional intelligence, and unshakable dedication, from the delicate touch that allays a patient's anxieties to the intricate medical procedures that save lives.

The varied abilities that are the foundation of providing great patient care are unraveled in this book, "Essential Nursing Skills," which dives into the core of nursing practice. We will travel through the core skills that all nurses need to have in the upcoming chapters, delving equally into the science and art of nursing.

This book will function as a thorough guide for both aspiring nurses and seasoned professionals, covering everything from developing critical thinking abilities to handling ethical dilemmas that frequently arise in healthcare settings, from mastering the art of effective communication to comprehending the nuances of medication administration. Through real-world examples, helpful advice, and evidence-based methods, readers will obtain priceless knowledge about the fundamental skills that characterize exceptional nursing.

Nursing is a calling, not just a career. It necessitates ongoing education, flexibility, and a strong desire to improve the lives of others. As we peruse the pages of "Essential Nursing Skills," let us embrace the essence of nursing: the steadfast dedication to providing patients with a holistic experience, the capacity for creativity when confronted with obstacles, and the significant influence that a knowledgeable and caring nurse can have on people as individuals, families, and communities.

Come along as we examine the fundamental abilities that turn regular people into exceptional nurses, one ability at a time, and help shape the future of healthcare.

CHAPTER ONE

ESSENTIALS OF PATIENT CARE

Crucial nursing Basic patient care abilities are essential to delivering high-quality medical care. These abilities are fundamental to nursing practice and have a major positive impact on patients' health.

A Notation:

To evaluate patients' conditions, identify changes, and react quickly to any signs of distress, nurses must possess keen observational skills.

Standard Hygiene

Comfort and infection prevention are enhanced when patients receive assistance with grooming, bathing, and other personal hygiene tasks.

Mobility Support:

Muscle atrophy and bedsores can be avoided by assisting patients in moving safely, whether it be through walking, changing positions in bed, or using assistive technology.

Administration of Medication:

Accurate medication administration, knowledge of dosage and possible side effects, and patient response monitoring are the duties of nurses.

Wound Care

To stop infections and encourage healing, wounds must be cleaned, dressed, and monitored properly.

Monitoring of Vital Signs:

Assessing a patient's general health requires routinely taking and interpreting vital signs, which include blood pressure, heart rate, respiration rate, and temperature.

Education of Patients:

Giving patients and their families knowledge about their illnesses, available treatments, and self-care encourages them to take an active role in their healing.

Crisis Intervention:

To ensure prompt action in emergencies, nurses should be trained in crisis management, CPR, and defibrillator use.

Control of Infections:

Comprehending and executing infection control measures aids in halting the transmission of illnesses in healthcare environments.

Recall that these abilities greatly enhance the overall patient experience and their road to recovery when applied with professionalism, kindness, and respect.

CHAPTER TWO

COMMUNICATION AND EMPATHY IN NURSING

Fundamental components of nursing practice, effective communication and empathy are essential for developing reliable patient relationships and delivering high-quality care.

Crucial Dialog in Nursing:

Simple and Direct Communication:

Information must be communicated, jargon must be

avoided, and patients must be made aware of their condition, course of treatment, and prescription drugs. Enhancing comprehension can be achieved by using simple language.

Listening intently:

Active listening to patients promotes trust and helps nurses better understand their needs, worries, and concerns. A holistic approach to care requires the ability to recognize nonverbal clues, which is another benefit of empathic listening.

Nonverbal Interaction:

Empathy and understanding can be expressed through gestures, facial expressions, and body language. Reassuring patients and demonstrating care and compassion can be accomplished by keeping eye contact and applying the proper touch.

Compassion and Emotional Assistance:

Nurses need to understand their patients' feelings and offer emotional support. Recognizing their emotions gives meaning to their experiences and reduces tension and anxiety.

Cultural Intelligence:

It is essential to understand and respect various cultural norms and values. By ensuring that communication is considerate of patients' cultural backgrounds, cultural competence fosters mutual respect and understanding.

Group Interaction:

Coordinated care depends on the healthcare team's ability to communicate effectively. To ensure seamless patient care, nurses must work in collaboration with other healthcare professionals and share critical information.

The Empathy of Nurses:

Considering the Patient in Totality:

Nurses with empathy take into account their patients' emotional, social, and psychological well-being in addition to their physical symptoms. Being aware of their entire circumstances facilitates the provision of individualized care.

Placing Oneself in the Situation of the Patient:

Empathy is putting oneself in the patient's shoes and trying to comprehend their thoughts, emotions, and worries. By adopting this perspective-taking approach, nurses can react to patients with empathy and comprehension.

Courtesy for dignity

Caring nurses respect and value their patients' autonomy while treating them with dignity and allowing them to participate in the decision-making process. The patient feels more in control and is in better health when this courteous approach is used.

Benevolent Touch:

Touching a patient appropriately, like holding their hand or giving them a reassuring pat, can reassure and show empathy. Touch can offer emotional support and a feeling of connectedness.

Keeping Emotional Limits in Check:

To avoid burnout, nurses need to be able to manage their emotional boundaries in addition to having empathy. Maintaining high-quality care requires striking a balance between professional detachment and sensitivity.

The cornerstones of nursing practice are empathy and effective communication. When nurses are skilled in these areas, they can help patients heal and feel better by offering not only the best physical care but also emotional and psychological support.

CHAPTER THREE

NURSING CLINICAL SKILLS

Essential nursing clinical skills are crucial for providing high-quality patient care and ensuring positive outcomes. Here are some key nursing clinical skills:

Evaluation of Patient:

To determine a patient's condition, track vital signs, and identify any changes in health status, nurses must perform comprehensive evaluations.

Administration of Medication:

Fundamental abilities include knowing how to calculate dosages, administering medications securely, and being aware of any possible negative effects.

Healing Care:

For a wound to heal and avoid complications, proper wound assessment, dressing changes, and infection prevention techniques are crucial.

Education of Patients:

Better understanding and compliance are encouraged when patients and their families are given information about their diseases, medications, and self-care methods.

Time Handling:

Nurses frequently balance a variety of patients and activities. Time management skills guarantee that every patient receives the right care.

Control of Infections:

To prevent illnesses linked to healthcare, be aware of and follow recommended hand hygiene, isolation measures, and sterilizing techniques.

Record-keeping:

For legal and continuity of care reasons, accurate and timely documentation of patient information—including assessments, actions, and outcomes—is essential.

Cooperation:

Effective teamwork among medical specialists, such as physicians, therapists, and other nurses, guarantees patient care that is well-coordinated and comprehensive.

Crisis Intervention:

Establishing priorities for work, staying composed under duress, and acting quickly in urgent or important situations.

Making Ethical Decisions:

To respect patients' rights and

make decisions that comply with both legal requirements and ethical standards, nurses must negotiate moral conundrums.

To hone these abilities and deliver top-notch nursing care, ongoing education, training, and practice are crucial.

CHAPTER FOUR

ANALYZATION AND SOLVING OF PROBLEMS

When navigating complex healthcare circumstances, nurses need to be able to think critically and solve problems. An explanation of these abilities within the nursing context:

Analytical Process:

Making well-reasoned decisions and doing objective information analysis are key components of critical thinking in nursing. It's about having an open mind, being observant, and having the capacity to weigh different viewpoints.

Clinical Evaluation:

It is the responsibility of nurses to evaluate patients' conditions, spot changes, and foresee any problems. Making accurate clinical decisions is aided by critical thinking.

Patient Involvement:

Nurses represent their patients' interests. They can assess available treatments thanks to critical thinking, which guarantees the highest quality of service.

Identification of the Problem:

It facilitates problem identification, awareness of underlying reasons, and successful resolution of challenges.

Practices Based on Evidence:

By using critical thinking skills, nurses may assess study results and make sure their practice is grounded in the most recent data. Nurses examine patient data to spot trends or outliers.

Patient Results:

Successful problem-solving enhances patient outcomes by resolving issues quickly and effectively.

Productivity:

By resolving administrative issues, nurses improve the efficiency of healthcare delivery as a whole.

Group Cooperation:

Collaboration is facilitated by problem-solving abilities, which makes healthcare teams more productive.

Identification of the Problem:

Problems can be clinical, administrative, or interpersonal; nurses are aware of them. Acquiring important information is essential to fully understanding the issue.

Idea generation:

Getting up with possible ideas fosters diversity of thought and creativity. weighing options, weighing advantages and disadvantages, and selecting the best course of action.

Cause-Related Analysis:

To stop a recurrence, nurses look into adverse events and pinpoint the underlying causes. Nurses examine workflows to identify inefficiencies and make necessary adjustments for improved results.

Handling Conflicts:

Resolving conflicts amongst team members in the healthcare industry and maintaining a positive work atmosphere.

Problem-solving and critical thinking are the cornerstones of nursing practice. These abilities help nurses deliver the best possible care to patients, improve healthcare procedures, and promote productive teamwork. Using ongoing skill development, nurses make a substantial contribution to the safety and quality of healthcare provision.

CHAPTER FIVE

TECHNICAL SKILLS FOR NURSING

Technical nursing abilities are necessary to deliver excellent patient care. These abilities include a broad spectrum of duties and operations that nurses carry out regularly.

Monitoring of Vital Signs:

Nurses must possess the necessary skills to measure and interpret vital signs, including blood pressure, heart rate, respiration rate, and temperature.

Administration of Medication:

Nurses must provide medications to patients, which involves being aware of the dosage, the best ways to administer it, and any possible side effects.

Intravenous Treatment (IV):

This entails setting up and maintaining intravenous lines for the delivery of blood products, medicines, and fluids.

Healing Care:

Infection control, wound assessment and dressing, and wound promotion are all areas in which nurses need to be experts.

Evaluation of Patient:

To create appropriate treatment plans, skilled nurses perform thorough assessments of patients that include social, psychological, and physical components.

Using a catheter

When necessary, nurses should be skilled in the insertion and maintenance of urinary catheters.

Exams for diagnosis:

To make sure patients are comfortable and ready for diagnostic procedures including blood tests, MRIs, X-rays, and ECGs, nurses frequently help.

Control of Ventilators:

Accuracy in ventilator management is vital for critical care nurses caring for patients experiencing discomfort.

Emergency Response:

To successfully tackle crises, nurses must be trained in both Advanced Cardiovascular Life Support (ACLS) and Basic Life Support (BLS).

Education of Patients:

Nurses provide details on medical illnesses, treatments, and self-care strategies to patients and their families.

Record-keeping:

Ensuring easy interaction among healthcare practitioners and preserving patient history depend heavily on prompt and accurate record-keeping.

Pain Control:

To assess and manage patients' pain, nurses frequently combine non-pharmacological approaches, physical therapy, and medication.

These technical abilities enable nurses to deliver patient-centered, comprehensive care when paired with empathy and skillful communication.

www.ingramcontent.com/pod-product-compliance
Lightning Source LLC
Chambersburg PA
CBHW072224290526
45794CB00007B/2884